better nutrition *magazine* presents

PREGNANCY

by CATHY CARLSON-RINK, ND

better nutrition healthy living guide

Published by:
Active Interest Media, Inc.
300 N. Continental Blvd., Suite 650
El Segundo, CA 90245

This booklet is part of the *Better Nutrition Healthy Living Guide* series. For more information, visit www.betternutrition.com. Better Nutrition magazine is available at fine natural health stores throughout the United States. Design by Aline Design: Bellingham, Wash.

PREGNANCY

CONTENTS

better nutrition healthy living guide

Chapter One
Preconception

Contemplating pregnancy is an exciting process for a family looking forward to welcoming a new life. But it's not all about nursery colors and baby names—growing a baby is hard work, and it comes with very specific nutritional demands. In fact, a woman's nutrition before and during pregnancy can have long-term effects not only on the child, but also on the woman herself.

Most of us think of pregnancy as a 9-month experience, but it is more accurate to view it as a childbearing year. The three months before pregnancy should be used to prepare the body to host a new life; the month following delivery is when the mother recovers from childbirth and begins to nourish her newborn. Research continues to show us that the nutritional status at the time of conception and in the first trimester, when all the fetus' organs are formed, sets the stage for a healthy pregnancy and a healthy baby.

Preconception Care

Before becoming pregnant, both partners should work to optimize their health. This entails addressing any current health issues and also changing any habits that don't contribute to a healthy pregnancy. Kicking lifetime habits is not easy, but it's much easier to tackle them before pregnancy than waiting until you see the two blue lines. Did you know that, even though it's universally accepted that smoking during pregnancy is terrible for the growing baby, only one in four women who try to quit when they're actually pregnant are successful?

There are plenty of reasons for a couple to take this time to improve health. Here are just a few:

- Optimizing fertility
- Improving nutritional stores
- Lowering toxic load
- Supporting proper detoxification and elimination
- Making healthy lifestyle changes that will serve you well as parents

The Association for the Promotion of Preconception Care conducted a study that shows the effectiveness of improving health prior to conception. In the study, 367 couples completed a program of improved nutrition and detoxification. Fifty-nine percent of the couples had a history of reproductive problems: 37 percent suffered infertility, 38 percent experienced miscarriages, 3 percent had had a stillbirth, and 15 percent gave birth to babies with low birth weights. Of the male partners, 42 percent had issues with sperm quality. After finishing the program laid out by the researchers, 89 percent of couples carried a pregnancy to term—including 86 percent of the couples with infertility problems. All babies were healthy and none required transfer to special care units.

Correct Nutritional Deficiencies

Nutrient deficiencies have been linked to infertility, repeat miscarriage, pregnancy complications, and low birth-weight infants. Evidence shows the mother's nutritional status around or before conception is the factor most strongly associated with healthy birth weight and head circumference.

Fertility Foods

Certain foods can actually improve fertility. A study of 17,500 women in the Nurse's Health Study revealed that fertility rates improved by eating a diet

- high in monounsaturated fat;
- low in trans fats;
- higher in vegetable protein (like beans and nuts);
- high in complex carbohydrates, including whole grains, fruits and vegetables; and
- high in full-fat dairy products.

Plant-based iron foods and iron supplements were also shown to decrease infertility (it's important to note that the same findings don't apply to iron from red meat). This study showed that women who took plant-based iron supplements during their pregnancy have a 40 percent reduction in infertility related to ovulation.

Antioxidants and vitamin B6 have been shown to improve luteal phase defect, a condition that causes infertility and miscarriage due to low progesterone in the second half of the menstrual cycle. Vitamins C and E and glutathione were found to be lower in women with a luteal phase defect. Women receiving 750 mg of vitamin C daily versus placebo improved their levels of progesterone and estrogen and had a higher pregnancy rate compared to placebo.

In addition, high levels the hormone prolactin, which can be increased by stress, excessive exercise, and low blood sugar, suppresses ovulation. Vitamin B6 reduces the levels of prolactin, which in turn encourages ovulation and progesterone production.

Balance Hormones

There has been a dramatic rise of estrogen-like synthetic chemicals (called xenoestrogens) in our environment. These estrogens are also called hormone or endocrine disrupters, as they can mimic or block natural hormones. Xenoestrogens are found in pesticides, plastics, and even tap water. In addition, many of the processed foods we eat stimulate estrogen receptors, which creates estrogen dominance in many women. This estrogen overload results in increased rates of fibrocystic breast disease, premenstrual syndrome, ovarian cysts, endometriosis, and infertility.

Strategies to Maintain Healthy Hormonal Balance

1. ***Reduce the Stimulation of Estrogen Receptors***
    - Eliminate sugar, soda pop, white flour, and refined foods.
    - Reduce caffeine-containing foods such as coffee, tea, and chocolate.
    - Avoid alcohol.

2. ***Remove Sources of Estrogen***
    - Eat organic food to reduce pesticide exposure.
    - Store and heat food in glass to reduce exposure to the xenoestrogens in soft plastics.
    - Drink filtered water; to avoid hormones and pesticide residues are in tap water.
    - Maintain your proper weight to reduce fat storage of environmental estrogens.
    - Avoid rapid weight loss, which releases toxins into your system.
    - Avoid conventional sources of dairy and meat which can contain hormones.

3. ***Improve Liver and Digestive Function***
    - The liver breaks down the hormones and releases them in the digestive tract for elimination. If you are constipated, the hormones are reabsorbed and re-formed, throwing off the hormonal balance again.
    - Eat liver-loving foods such as beets, artichokes, lemons, garlic, and onions.
    - Eat bitter foods and herbs to stimulate bile production, which releases hormones into the digestive tract.
    - Stimulate effective elimination from the digestive tract with a high-fiber diet and add ground flaxseeds, a source of healthy phytoestrogens.
    - Support detoxification pathways with an herbal detoxification formula, such as Floressence. *NOTE: Do not attempt to conceive while on a detoxification program.*
    - Support optimum digestion with digestive enzymes and probiotics
    - Help eliminate wastes via sweat by exercising, hydrotherapy treatments, and saunas.

Reduce Your Toxic Load

Toxins aren't good for anyone, but fetuses and young babies are particularly vulnerable to exposure to hazardous chemicals and heavy metals, as their brains and organs are developing rapidly. Toxic substances can disrupt correct signals for normal development. If a mother is exposed to harmful substances, she can potentially transfer those toxins to the baby via the placenta or breast milk. Choosing infant formula is not the solution, as besides being processed and packaged, it is also high in toxins.

In addition to the previous suggestions to improve liver and digestive function, which will help rid toxins from the body, women who want to get pregnant should take these steps as well.

- Quit smoking and avoid alcohol beverages.
- Avoid use of pesticides in the home and garden.
- Avoid exposure to solvents such as paints, non-water-based glues, furniture strippers, gasoline fumes, and nail polish.
- Avoid dry cleaners and dry cleaned clothes.
- Eat low on the food chain, avoiding large amounts of animal fats and high-fat dairy products that can store chemical residues.
- Avoid fish with high mercury and PCB levels, such as swordfish and shark.
- Eat organic food whenever possible.
- Achieve your optimal weight.

It is very important to maintain a normal weight prior to pregnancy. Studies link obesity with a tenfold increase in maternal blood pressure, a 10 percent increase in gestational diabetes, more difficult deliveries that result in higher rates of induction and c-section, and increased risks of congenital defects, especially neural tube defects.

Get Off The Pill

If you have been using hormonal birth control, you should be off it for at least six months before conceiving. The birth control pill causes deficiencies in folic acid, B6 (which can lead to lower progesterone production), vitamin E, magnesium and zinc. Especially important is the effect on folic acid, which is necessary for preventing neural tube defects like spina bifida, and it takes the body six months to restore normal levels after discontinuing birth control. A multivitamin can help mitigate the effects of the pill.

Learn Fertility Awareness

During the preconception time, learn about natural family planning. This includes recognizing signs of fertility by monitoring your basal body temperature and changes in cervical mucus. When you track this information for a couple of months, you'll learn your optimal time to try to conceive. For more information on fertility awareness, read the book *Taking Charge of Your Fertility* (Collins Living, 2006) by Toni Weschler, MPH. Use barrier methods while you are learning fertility awareness.

Give up Bad Habits

Smoking, alcohol and street drugs have been shown to negatively affect the health of the sperm, egg and fetus. Since the crucial time for cell division and formation of the baby is in the first 12 weeks of pregnancy, it is best to avoid these substances for several months prior to conception. Smoking during pregnancy leads to lower birth-weight infants, higher rates of prematurity, congenital malformations, and higher infant death rates.

Alcohol consumption by the mother has been linked to fetal alcohol syndrome. Thresholds of minimum amounts that can be consumed safely have not been established. We now know that a child can also have subtler physical or mental deficiencies from alcohol exposure without having an actual diagnosis of Fetal Alcohol Syndrome.

In addition, alcohol consumption leads to nutritional deficiencies in the mother due to reduced appetite, decreased absorption of nutrients from the digestive tract, and increase of urinary excretion of vitamins and minerals. Folic acid and zinc status is particularly affected.

In men, both alcohol and tobacco reduce sperm counts and increases the number of damaged sperm. Alcohol is a testicular toxin that causes structural loss of tubules and sperm cells and reduces the synthesis and secretion of testosterone.

Caffeine has been linked to a higher rate of miscarriage. In a recent Swedish study, women who consumed more than five cups of coffee daily were twice as likely to have a miscarriage than those who consumed less than one cup.

Exercise

Women who remain physically active during pregnancy have been found to have shorter deliveries with fewer complications. Research shows that women who exercise have significantly fewer medical interventions (induced labors, episiotomies, and cesarean sections, for example) than those who do not. Their babies suffer less distress during labor and after delivery. Walking, swimming, exercise classes in water, and yoga are good pregnancy exercises, especially for those with a history of inactivity. Pregnancy is not a time to start a new, vigorous training program. Pregnancy is time to maintain what you have gained in your pre-pregnancy fitness program.

Substances That Reduce Fertility

- Caffeine
- Commercial Dairy
- Sugar and Processed Foods
- Chemicals in Plastics
- Trans Fats
- Pesticides
- Xenoestrogens

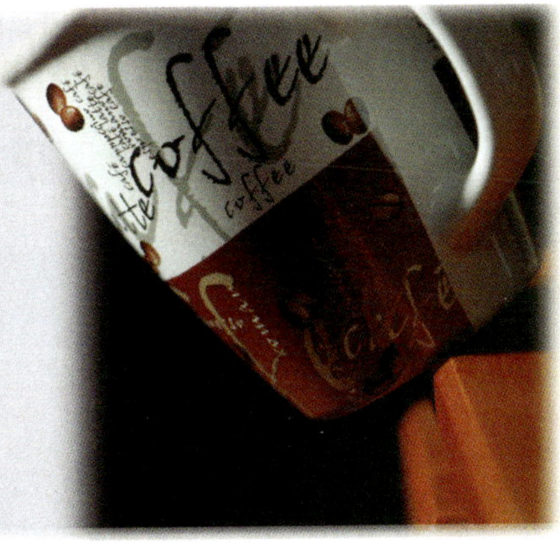

Reduce Miscarriage Risk

Miscarriage is devastating for a mother and her family. However, as hard as it is, many miscarriages happen for a reason. Unless they're recurrent, miscarriages may be nature's screening system to ensure only healthy babies are born. Of course, this does not make it any easier to experience. Many women question what they could have done differently to avoid miscarriage. The reality is that 60 to 80 percent of miscarriages are genetic, and there is nothing you can do to prevent them. An interesting study looked at things that might influence miscarriage that can serve as a guide for possibly decreasing miscarriage risk, but unfortunately there's no way to avoid it altogether. The study interviewed 6,000 women about their pregnancy histories and found some trends.

Factors that decreased risk:

- Taking vitamins, particularly iron and folic acid, reduced risk by 50 percent.
- Consumption of fresh fruits, vegetables and dairy products by 50 percent.
- Positive emotional health reduced risk by 60 percent.
- History of already having had a live birth reduced risk by 40 percent.
- Nausea in first trimester reduced risk by 70 percent.

Factors that increased risk:

- Maternal age between 35 and 39 years compared to those aged 25 to 29.
- Low pre-pregnancy weight.
- History of miscarriage.
- Infertility or taking more than one year to conceive.
- Stressful or demanding job.
- Feeling stressed, depressed, or overwhelmed.
- Regular alcohol consumption.
- There was no correlation found with prolonged sitting, standing, or heavy lifting.

Chapter Two
Nutrition Basics

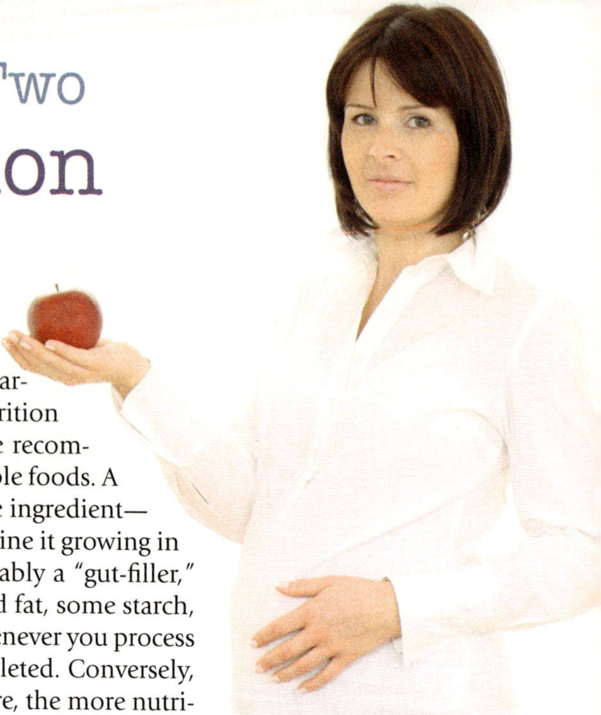

In a complex world of food choices, I narrow my basic nutrition advice down to a simple recommendation: Eat real, whole foods. A whole food has only one ingredient—itself. If you cannot imagine it growing in the earth, then it is probably a "gut-filler," providing calories, rancid fat, some starch, sugar, and little else. Whenever you process a food, nutrients are depleted. Conversely, the closer we eat to nature, the more nutrient-dense the foods will be. Whole foods contain the complete set of nutrients needed for your body to be able to process them. Nutrient-dense foods pack a lot of punch because they are rich in important vitamins and minerals. This is especially vital in pregnancy, because even though pregnancy only requires 300 extra calories, it calls for many more nutrients are required. During pregnancy, the need for protein, essential fats, calcium, magnesium, iron, and zinc increase dramatically.

Eat Organic And Local

Local foods are the freshest and tastiest, and because they are picked ripe they have a higher nutrient content. Because they are not shipped long distances, they have fewer chemicals to preserve them. Organic foods have a high nutrient content and they reduce the mother and baby's exposure to toxins (pesticides, herbicides, fungicides, hormones, and genetically modified organisms).

Eat a Variety Foods

Every food has a slightly different nutrient make-up, so variety—even within a food group—helps decrease the risk of nutritional deficiencies. This also reduces our chance of food allergies, as there is less chance of an immune response if our body does not see a food repetitively. Eat lots of different colors, as the dark pigmented foods are rich in antioxidants and phytonutrients. Eat raw, as these foods are full of enzymes to aid digestion. Fermented foods such as yogurt and miso are pre-digested, so there is less work required by the digestive tract, which will help with nausea and vomiting during pregnancy.

Quality Protein

Pregnancy is a time of growth, making amino acids and protein especially important. Amino acids are the building blocks for the growth and maintenance of bones, teeth, organs, and tissues. Amino acids help regulate body processes to produce enzymes and hormones, ensure proper immune function, and transport oxygen.

A woman's need for protein increases to 50 grams daily when she becomes pregnant. To meet protein needs, try to have a small amount with each meal. Focus on organic plant sources of protein to avoid exposure to pesticides, hormones, and other chemicals that can be found in nonorganic meat and dairy. Interestingly, those who eat more beans and nuts as a protein source have higher fertility rate. The healthiest protein sources include legumes, whole grains, raw nuts and seeds, organic yogurt with live cultures, tofu, cold-water wild fish like salmon, and free-range or certified organic meats.

Foundational Fats

Fats provide essential fatty acids (omega-3 and -6) needed for optimum reproduction and cell membranes for the placenta. Fats are needed for the absorption, storage, and circulation of fat-soluble vitamins A, D, E, and K. Cultures that consume a higher amount of cold-water fish rich in omega 3s have less preterm labor, less growth problems for the fetus, and a lower incidence of preeclampsia. Because the placenta is rich in cell membranes that require essential fatty acids, it is critical they are present in the diet around the time of conception.

While many people are aware of the role of fish and fish oil, specifically omega-3, in infant brain and visual development, people rarely look at the fats they are consuming in their diet overall. Omega-3 fatty acids need to be balanced with omega-6 fatty acids to be most effective. Supplementation with DHA (an omega-3) by itself can reduce the amounts of the omega-6 fats GLA and arachidonic acid. GLA is needed for ensuring sufficient birth weight, increasing breast milk supply, and reducing risk of insulin resistance. Arachidonic acid is important for infant brain development and function. Most people do not consume enough omega-3 fatty acids, and although omega-6 fatty acids are present in the diet, they are easily destroyed by food processing. Most studies show fat quality, as opposed to fat quantity, ultimately predicts risks. A diet high in essential fatty acids along with fruit, vegetables, and whole grains is the best. Limit your amount of saturated fat and cholesterol, as they tend to be overconsumed. However, they are necessary for making reproductive hormones and are a good source for arachidonic acid. Pick quality sources such as organic yogurt, butter, eggs and 4 ounce servings of meats.

Essential fatty acids are destroyed by heat and light, so eat them raw rather than in the form of a dietary supplement. Oils should be cold pressed and stored in dark glass bottles. I recommend Udo's Oil DHA 3•6•9 Blend for dressings, smoothies, and sauces. Natural sources of omega 3 include flaxseed, soybeans, walnut, pumpkinseed, dark leafy green vegetables, and cold-water fish like salmon, trout, tuna, mackerel, ocean perch, Alaskan pollock, and arctic char. Omega-6 sources include sesame, sunflower, and evening primrose oil.

On the other side of the equation, we have the bad fats, which are trans fats. Trans fatty acids lower essential fatty acid levels in both mothers and babies during both pregnancy and breastfeeding. Avoid trans fats whenever possible by avoiding hydrogenated oils and reading labels carefully.

Carbohydrates: The More Complex The Better

Carbohydrates provide our main source of energy. The most basic carbohydrate is glucose (sugar). Complex carbohydrates help regulate the metabolism of protein and fat, and they provide fiber for blood sugar regulation and effective elimination from the digestive tract. Higher fiber diets are linked with lower rates of gestational diabetes and preeclampsia.

Unfortunately, most people consume simple carbohydrates in the form of crackers, breads, pasta, cake and cookies. These refined carbohydrates have been stripped of their fiber, so they cause a roller coaster effect on the blood sugar. America's consumption of simple carbohydrates may be one of the reasons for our dramatic increases in obesity and diabetes.

When the low fat diet first became popular, manufacturers introduced fat-free products high in simple carbs. Consumption of refined white-flour pasta, muffins, and crackers skyrocketed, along with fruit drinks and soda pop. So how does this affect pregnancy? Whenever you eat a refined carbohydrate, such as a white-flour muffin, there is minimal fiber. As a result, sugar and starch move rapidly into the bloodstream, resulting in high blood sugar. Glucose is also one of the easiest things to cross the placenta, so the baby gets more glucose and, consequently, is likely to be born at a higher birth weight, even when a mother's weight gain may be normal. My general rule for patients is to avoid anything white (sugar and flour).

Sources of complex carbohydrates include vegetables, whole grains, legumes, and whole fruit.

Power Pregnancy Foods

Dark Green & Leafy Vegetables

These are truly nature's fast foods, as they cook quickly—and many can even be eaten raw. They are the perfect pregnancy food, full of vital nutrients such as calcium, magnesium, B vitamins, iron, trace minerals, folic acid, and vitamin K. They are also great sources of antioxidants and carotenes.

Add more of the following to your diet: kale, watercress, beet greens, bok choy, Chinese (Napa) cabbage, collard greens, dandelion greens, endive, mustard greens, Swiss chard, and turnip greens.

Yellow and Orange Vegetables

Rich in carotenes, yellow and orange veggies contain potent antioxidants, boost immune function, aid the growth and repair of tissue, reduce ultraviolet damage to skin, and support eye and skin health.

Good choices include carrots, yams, pumpkin, squash, and sweet potatoes.

Broccoli and Cabbage Family

High intake of cruciferous vegetables like broccoli and cabbage is important for immune function. These veggies are high in indols and carotenoids, which have been proven to possess anti-cancer properties. Broccoli is also a great source of calcium, vitamin C, potassium, and iron. Some mothers need to avoid this vegetable group in the first three months of nursing. It can increase gas and colic in the infant, due to digestive immaturity.

Other members of the cruciferous family: Brussels sprouts, kale, bok choy, collards, turnips, mustard greens, kohlrabi, and watercress.

Dark Pigmented Berries

High in antioxidants and rich in fiber, potassium, vitamin C, and flavonoids known as anthocyanins, berries boost the immune system and reduce free-radical damage and inflammation. They help with collagen formation, eyesight, and circulation. Oxidative damage (from free radicals) has been linked to gestational diabetes and preeclampsia, so eating a diet high in antioxidants makes sense. Also, berries in combination with fermented milk products like yogurt have been shown to reduce the incidence of urinary tract infections that can cause kidney infections and term labor.

Food sources include rosehips, blackberries, blueberries, raspberries, cranberries and strawberries.

Nuts And Seeds

Nuts and seeds are high in essential fatty acids, vitamin E, and concentrated protein. Essential fatty acids found in nuts and seeds help influence cellular strength, balance hormones, protect nerves, and reduce inflammation. They are also concentrated sources of vitamins and minerals like calcium, magnesium, and zinc. Consume raw or as cold pressed, unrefined vegetable oils

Cashews, almonds, walnuts, sunflower seeds, flax seeds, sesame seeds are good choices.

Plain, Organic Yogurt With Live Cultures

This fermented food enhances digestion and is a great source of complete protein, calcium, B12, potassium, and zinc. Both prebiotics (food for probiotics that aids in absorption of calcium), and probiotics (beneficial organisms for the digestive tract) are important. Probiotics have demonstrated the ability to enhance the immune system and aid in detoxification. Probiotics compete with yeast and "bad" bacteria to prevent urinary tract infections and yeast infections that can be more prevalent during pregnancy.

Spices

Unfortunately, sugar and salt are the main condiments in North America. Conversely, 50 percent of the foods in the East Indian diet include health-promoting spices such as turmeric. Many spices are high in antioxidants, have antimicrobial properties, and stimulate healthy digestion and circulation. Spices should be non-irradiated to maintain the therapeutic potential of the substance. Many culinary herbs have healing properties. Curcumin, found in turmeric and mustard, is a potent anti-inflammatory.

Whole Grains

Whole grains are superior to refined grains because they have more protein, fiber, B vitamins, calcium, iron, and vitamin E. B vitamins are key, as they are necessary for the release of energy from carbohydrates, protein, and fat.

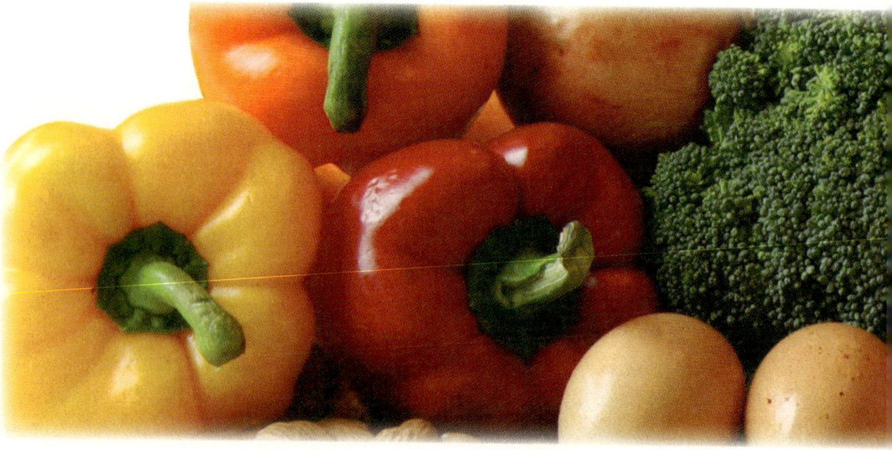

Sources of whole grains include whole wheat, brown rice, barley, steel cut oats, corn, buckwheat, rye, millet, quinoa, spelt, amaranth, and teff.

Legumes

Legumes like beans are staples around the world but are eaten comparatively rarely in North America. They are high in protein, complex carbohydrates, fiber, iron, B vitamins, folic acid, potassium and magnesium, and low in fat. Regular consumption has shown to stabilize blood sugar, reduce obesity and high blood pressure, and relieve constipation. They are also a rich source of antioxidants. The darker the pigment, the higher the antioxidant activity.

Add these legumes to your diet: black beans, pinto beans, chickpeas, lima beans, fava beans, mung beans, aduki beans, soybeans, white beans, cranberry beans, lentils, peas, and green beans.

Cold-Water Fish

Cold-water fish is high in omega-3 fatty acids and vitamin D. Due to high mercury content, avoid shark and swordfish. Salmon has been shown to have the lowest levels of toxins and heavy metals.

Free-Range, Organic Eggs

Eggs are rich in protein, zinc, and vitamins A, D, E, and B12. Eggs are also a great source of choline and betaine, both involved in the process of methylation that reduces homocysteine levels. Elevated homocysteine levels have been linked to infertility and complications in pregnancy. Choline is also necessary for the structure and function of cell membranes and for the production of brain chemicals to boost memory and concentration. Animal studies have demonstrated that choline taken from mid-pregnancy to birth improved learning and memory recall in the newborn and that the effects were lifelong.

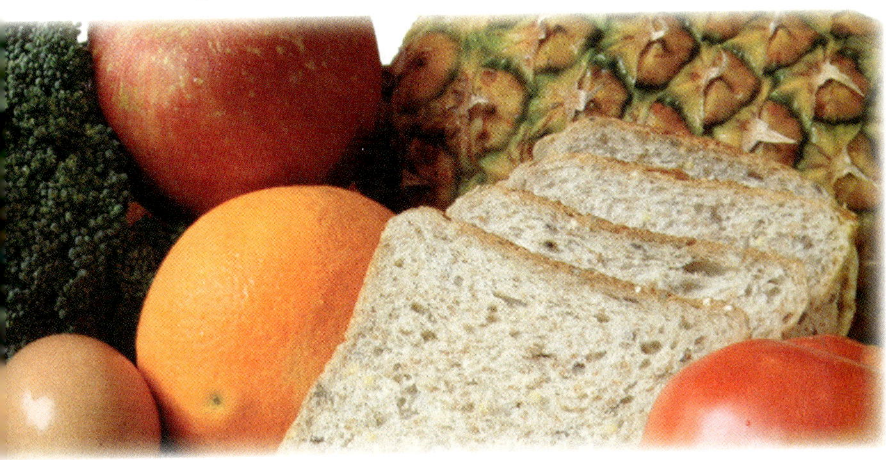

Chapter Three
Common Complaints

The body is very smart. During pregnancy it makes physiological adaptations to accommodate the growing baby and to prepare the body for labor. The uterus increases its size by 500 to 1,000 times. Lung function, cardiac output, kidney function, the immune system, and metabolism are all boosted during pregnancy. The availability of nutrients improves, partly because the hormone progesterone acts on the digestive tract to slow the time it takes food to travel, thus increasing the time for absorption.

Sometimes we experience the effects of these changes with discomforts. For example, blood volume dramatically increases to compensate for blood loss at birth. However, this results in a drop in blood pressure, which can contribute to dizziness and headaches. Increased blood volume can also increase sinus congestion and cause bleeding gums and noses. To fully enjoy your pregnancy, you need ways to lessen its inherent discomforts. Here are some suggestions for dealing with some of the most common complaints.

Nausea And Vomiting

There are many theories as to why women become nauseous during pregnancy, particularly in the first trimester. The sharp rise in hormones that the liver is required to process, along with sluggish digestion due to progesterone, could contribute to nausea. Morning sickness may actually serve a purpose. Some experts believe it causes strong aversions to protect the baby from harmful compounds. It also stimulates placenta development, reduces the woman's energy expenditure, and actually increases nutrient intake in some cases. The most important thing is to manage your symptoms and consult a health care professional if your nausea and vomiting is prolonged or excessive or you have concerns about dehydration.

Here are some suggestions to help ease nausea:

- Eat small frequent meals; nausea seems to be worse when the stomach is too full or too empty or blood sugar is low.
- Reduce your saturated fats, as they increase the severity of nausea and vomiting.
- Get enough sleep and relaxation. Fatigue and stress make nausea worse.

- Stay hydrated by drinking liquids between meals.
- Eat easy-to-digest foods such as smoothies, soup, steamed veggies, fruit, crackers, toast, fermented foods like miso and yogurt, and foods high in digestive enzymes like pineapple.
- B6 (30 mg/day) can reduce the severity of morning sickness, according to two double-blind trials.
- A randomized, double-blind, placebo-controlled trial found ginger (250 mg 4x/day) significantly reduced nausea and vomiting compared to placebo.
- 11 studies found acupressure/acupuncture to a specific point on the wrist was effective at reducing symptoms. Sea bands are one option available in providing pressure to this point.

Heartburn

During pregnancy, the growing baby and uterus displaces the intestines and stomach upward. In addition, the digestive system tone is decreased, resulting in gastric reflux (heartburn). Women who have heartburn should take the following steps,

- Eat small meals and avoid lying down for at least an hour after eating.
- Avoid spicy and greasy foods.
- Eat fruits high in digestive enzymes (grapefruit, papaya, pineapple); consider taking a digestive enzyme supplement.
- Take liquid calcium/magnesium (1 teaspoon before meals) to coat and protect the esophagus; I recommend the Flora brand.

Leg Cramps And Restless Legs

Leg cramps and restless legs usually occur in the third trimester of pregnancy. During this time, the baby needs additional bone-building nutrients for its skeleton and to build iron stores for the first six months of life. If the mother does not have enough of these nutrients in her diet, they are extracted from her stores. Leg cramps and restless legs are symptoms that the mother is not getting enough vital nutrients to protect her own body. Fortunately this is easily corrected with diet and supplementation.

The most common cause of leg cramps is a magnesium deficiency. Supplement with 1 to 2 Tbsp. of Liquid Calcium/Magnesium in a 1:1 ratio at bedtime. If leg cramps do not resolve, add in additional magnesium (up to 500 mg/day). The next two nutrient deficiencies that can cause leg cramps are vitamin E & iron. To ease restless legs take 30 mg of iron and 400 IU of vitamin E daily.

Constipation

Constipation is more common in pregnancy due to sluggish digestion and compression of the intestines. The increase in progesterone acts to decrease the tone, motility and secretions of the digestive tract. It is aggravated by poorly absorbed iron supplements. I suggest the following:

- Drink eight to 10 glasses of filtered water daily.
- Eat foods high in fiber (whole fruits and veggies, oat bran and flaxseed, for example).
- 1 Tbsp. of ground flaxseed in 8 oz. of water, followed by another 8 oz of water brings quick resolution to constipation.
- Stimulate bile secretion to encourage a bowel movement with lemon juice, artichokes, beets, and turmeric.
- Avoid constipating foods: meat, white flour, excessive dairy, pizza, and unripe bananas.
- Exercise to increase the motility of the intestines and stimulate a bowel movement.
- Take probiotics. People with constipation are often deficient in friendly organisms in their gut. Lactobacillus strains encourage peristalsis, the rhythmic movement that helps move the contents of the intestines for efficient elimination.

Varicose Veins And Hemorrhoids

As the baby grows, it is harder for blood to return from the lower body—leading to varicose veins and hemorrhoids. Take these steps to avoid these problems:

- Wear support hose to compress enlarged vessels and decrease pain.
- Elevate legs and exercise daily to improve circulation.
- Eat 1 cup of blueberries daily to increase intake of vitamin C and bioflavonoids, which support blood vessel strength.
- Resolve constipation, which exacerbates hemorrhoids.
- Use witch hazel compresses topically to reduce swelling of hemorrhoids.

Lower-Leg Swelling

Leg swelling is typically not serious, unless severe, but it can be very uncomfortable. Again it is due to the decreased venous and lymphatic return from the lower body. Try the following:

- Elevate legs when at rest to encourage blood to return to the heart.
- Walk, as the contraction of the lower leg muscles creates a pumping action on the blood vessels, enhancing circulation.
- Drink plenty of water.
- Decrease the swelling by taking vitamin B6 (50 mg/day) and Salus dandelion juice.

Chapter Four

Preventing Complications

In modern obstetrics, many incredible advances have been made to save mothers' and babies' lives. However, preeclampsia (previously known as toxemia in pregnancy) and preterm labor continue to cause complications in pregnancy. In fact, over the last forty years, the number of women affected by preeclampsia has remained unchanged. Once these diseases develop, effective treatment is limited. Although the diagnosis of gestational diabetes remains controversial, it also does not respond very well to treatment. Therefore, the best approach is to take steps to prevent these diseases in the first place.

Please note, once these conditions are diagnosed they require ongoing care and sometimes urgent care from an obstetrical care provider. This ensures the safety of both mother and baby.

These three diseases are an intertwining story of similar causes and risk factors. Elevated homocysteine levels, free-radical damage, and nutrient deficiencies contribute to all three. Each disease can increase the risk of developing one of the others. For example, if you have gestational diabetes, you have an increased risk of preeclampsia and preterm labor. If you have preeclampsia, you are at risk of having a preterm birth.

The Homocysteine Connection

Plasma levels are 30 to 60 percent lower during pregnancy than at other times. The lowest levels occur in the second trimester. This may be a physiological adaptation during pregnancy mediated by hormonal changes. Research shows that it may have a role in keeping the body balanced during pregnancy. Keeping homocysteine levels normal is essential to maintaining a healthy pregnancy.

Measuring homocysteine levels can tell us about methylation function in the body. Methylation is a chemical process in the body that is needed for formation of hormones and insulin, production of cellular energy, and synthesis and repair of genetic material, including in the developing baby. Methylation also helps detoxify heavy metals and mobilizes and eliminates fat and cholesterol. If homocysteine is low, then methylation is working properly.

High homocysteine levels have been linked with neural tube defects (like spina bifida), childhood leukemia, Down Syndrome, birth defects, gestational diabetes, preeclampsia, male and female infertility, repeated miscarriage, preterm labor, and placental abruption. Measuring homocysteine is an effective tool for prevention, as it can be elevated before the onset of disease symptoms. For example, elevated homocysteine in the first trimester increases the risk fourfold of developing preeclampsia.

Folic Acid is Not The Whole Story

Many women are aware of the recommendation to take folic acid during the three months before conception to prevent neural tube defects like spina bifida. However, folic acid, B12, B6, betaine, and choline (found in eggs and in lecithin) are all needed to ensure that methylation occurs properly. In fact, B12 has been shown to be even more effective in protecting against spina bifida than folic acid. Supplementing with folic acid alone can also mask a B12 deficiency and is not effective at preventing other diseases associated with high homocysteine levels. Studies indicate there is a fourfold increase in preterm labor with elevated homocysteine levels. Some studies show there is a 60 percent increase risk with a B12 deficiency and a 50 percent increase with a B6 deficiency, but no link with folic acid. The combination of B6, B12, and folic acid has been found effective at reducing homocysteine levels.

Antioxidants

Free-radical damage is another piece of the puzzle. Free radicals are unstable molecules that can damage cell membranes, proteins, DNA, contributing to various diseases. Oxidative stress as a result of free radical generation has also been demonstrated in gestational diabetes, preeclampsia, and preterm labor.

Vitamin C

Vitamin C is a powerful water-soluble antioxidant that helps boost the immune system, lay down and maintain connective tissue, heal wounds, strengthen blood vessels, aid iron absorption, and reduce allergic response. Vitamin C deficiencies have been linked with recurrent miscarriage, preterm labor, premature rupture of membranes, gestational diabetes, and preeclampsia. A double-blind, randomized trial of 126 women published in the *American Journal of Clinical Nutrition* showed that only 7.7 percent of women experienced premature rupture of membranes when taking 100 mg of vitamin C daily, versus 24.5 percent in the control group. In 2004 the *Journal of Reproductive Medicine* reported that women who consume less than 70 mg per day of vitamin C had fourfold increase risk of gestational diabetes. The people with the lowest blood levels of vitamin C had a twelvefold increased risk of gestational diabetes.

Vitamin E

Deficiency of vitamin E, a fat-soluble antioxidant and anti-inflammatory nutrient, has been linked to increased rates of miscarriage and low fertility in men. One of vitamin E's main roles may be in preventing miscarriage caused by autoimmune disease.

Grape Seed

Grape seed extract contains a powerful antioxidant and cell and tissue protector known as Oligomeric ProanthoCyanidin (OPC). OPCs are 20 times more powerful than vitamin C and 50 times more powerful than vitamin E in their ability to scavenge free radicals. They maintain the structure and integrity of the veins, arteries, and capillaries, ensuring efficient circulation. OPCs strengthen collagen by preventing enzymatic attack, free-radical destruction and excessive cross-linking.

Exercise And Stress Management

Exercise has shown to reduce oxidative stress by increasing free-radical scavengers and lowering low-density "bad" cholesterol. Taking time to relax not only reduces free radicals but also gives your body the rest it needs to restore and maintain optimum function.

Nutrient Deficiencies

Because of the increased nutritional demands in pregnancy, it is easier to become deficient in vital nutrients. Iron, calcium, magnesium, vitamin D, and zinc play a particular role in disease prevention in pregnancy.

Iron

Iron deficiency is the No. 1 deficiency in pregnancy and is often misdiagnosed and mistreated. For women in general, iron is the most common deficiency in the world. From the first period (menarche) to the last period (menopause), a woman's iron level is determined by the loss of the mineral during menstruation and pregnancy. Research shows only one in five fertile women starts her pregnancy with adequate iron levels. Women's iron requirements

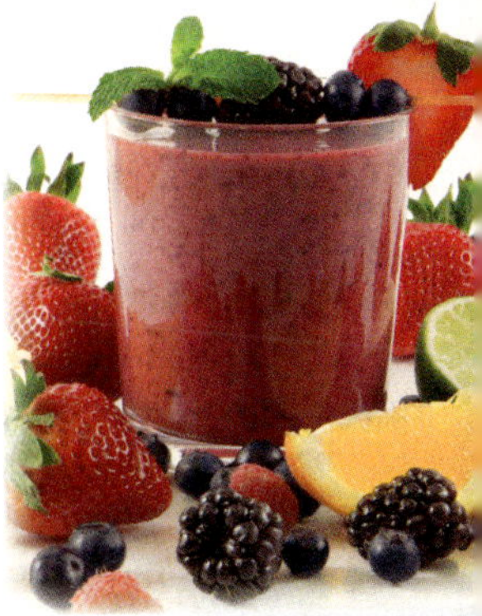

Antioxidant-rich Foods

Fruits

Blueberries

Blackberries

Cranberries

Strawberries

Vegetables

Kale

Spinach

Broccoli

Beets

Red Peppers

Spices

Oregano

Cinnamon

Sage

Peppermint

Thyme

Turmeric

double during pregnancy and, without proper diet and effective supplementation, iron stores can drop and continue to decline with each subsequent pregnancy. The key is to prevent the problem in the first place with adequate dietary intake and safe iron supplementation.

Adequate iron is needed for optimum fertility, proper placental development at the time of conception, efficient oxygen delivery to the baby, brain development in the baby, and formation of iron stores for the baby's first six months of life. Iron deficiency in pregnancy is linked with miscarriage, low birth weight, preterm labor, postpartum depression, and iron deficiency in infants.

Lab Testing: Iron deficiency Does Not Equal Anemia

Recent studies are showing that mild iron deficiency robs your body of optimum function well before anemia develops. In fact, iron deficiency effects cellular energy, detoxification, thyroid and heart function before there is any affect on the red blood cells. Iron is found in hemoglobin and carries oxygen to your tissues. Women feel exhausted due to low oxygen levels and lower thyroid and cell function. Anemia, low red blood cell count or low hemoglobin, will develop if iron deficiency is left unchecked long enough. Anemia develops when iron stores are almost completely depleted. This makes hemoglobin a poor screening test. A woman has to be deficient for a long time before anemia is detected. This requires more treatment and more severe symptoms have likely already developed. In addition, the hemoglobin measurement is more inaccurate in pregnancy because the rise of blood volume makes the blood more dilute. Serum ferritin and the size of the red blood cells are the most sensitive tests for detecting iron deficiency in pregnancy. Fertile women planning a pregnancy should have iron stores of 40–70 ug/l. If adequate stores are not present, low-dose supplementation is indicated.

Prevention is The Key

The safest option to prevent iron deficiency during pregnancy is with low-dose iron supplementation to help meet the recommended daily allowance.

Planning a pregnancy should include making sure you have adequate iron stores. Research shows 20 mg per day of iron helps four out of five women who have iron deficiency but have not been diagnosed with anemia. The Nurses' Health Study found that those who take plant-sourced iron supplements during the fertile years are 40 percent less likely to suffer from infertility related to ovulation.

Safe Iron Supplementation

Most women who have 15 mg of iron in their diets and 30 mg in a supplement are able to meet their requirement for iron in pregnancy. A

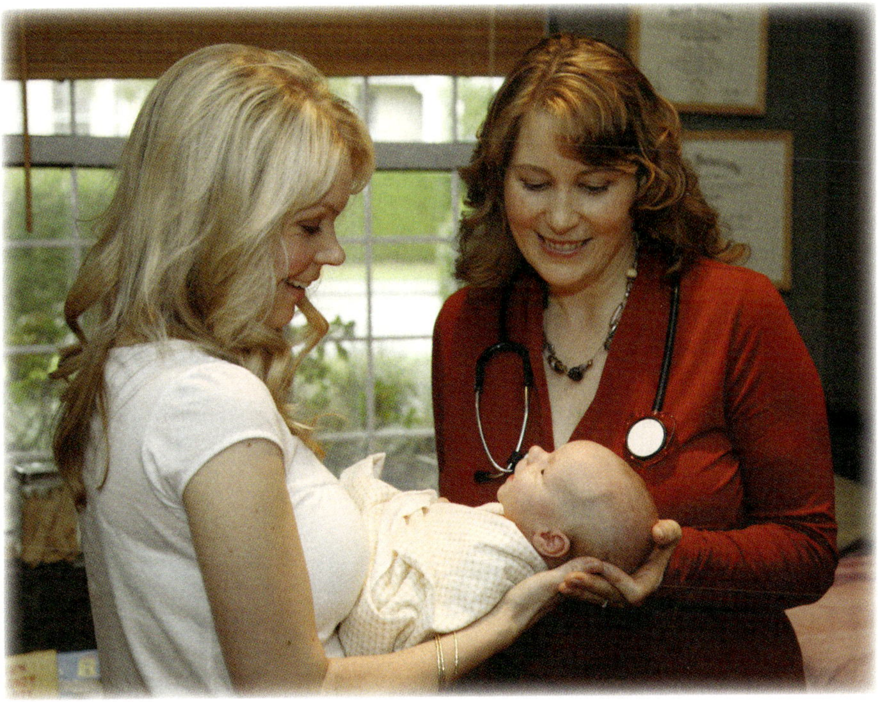

Dr. Carlson-Rink pictured with a happy and healthy patient.

2003 study from the *American Journal of Clinical Nutrition* showed that using a low-dose iron supplement of 20 mg per day from the 20th week of pregnancy through delivery reduced anemia and iron deficiency at delivery and postpartum without the side effects usually found with high-dose iron supplements such as digestive upset and constipation. Another study in the same journal that year found that taking 30 mg of iron in the first trimester was 76 percent effective in reducing low birth-weight babies even with women who had adequate iron levels. A third study compared taking a 30 mg iron supplement versus placebo during the second half of pregnancy and found that those who supplemented with iron did not develop anemia, compared to 14 percent in the placebo group. Pregnant mothers who took iron supplements returned to normal iron levels by six months postpartum, whereas it took two years for those women who did not.

High Doses of Iron Are a Concern

If you wait until you're anemic, you'll need higher doses of iron to correct the problem. High-dose iron supplements in pregnancy are very poorly tolerated, causing constipation and digestive upset. There's also a concern that doses of higher than 50 mg per day in pregnancy may be linked with high blood pressure in mothers, and with free-radical damage.

Surprisingly, high doses have also been found to increase the rate of low birth-weight babies and premature births, which are actually prevented with low-dose supplementation. Neither iron deficiency nor iron overload is beneficial to the body. Finding the balance with diet and low-dose supplementation is essential.

Calcium

Calcium is the main ingredient in bone and teeth and is needed for proper blood clotting and heart, nerve, and muscle function. Calcium deficiency has been linked with a higher incidence of preeclampsia. Higher levels of calcium are needed not only to build the infant's bones but to protect the mother's bones as well. Pregnancy can be protective against osteoporosis as long as the mother is well nourished.

For women who have grown up on processed food, insulin resistance has become a key risk factor for blood sugar imbalance during pregnancy.

Magnesium

Magnesium deficiency is one of the most common deficiencies in the Western world. A pregnant woman's needs increase to 350 mg per day, but the standard diet provides only about 165 mg per day. Magnesium works in tandem with calcium for heart, nerve, and muscle function. It is needed for bone strength, blood sugar regulation, and the operation of more than 300 enzymes, including those that break down and utilize fats, proteins, and carbohydrates.

Deficiencies in magnesium have been linked with preeclampsia, preterm labor, premature rupture of membranes, and nighttime leg cramps. A 2000 study in the *European Journal of Clinical Nutrition* found children born to mothers who ate a high-magnesium diet had higher bone masses at 8 years of age. Research shows 65 percent of those with insulin resistance syndrome are magnesium deficient. For women who have grown up on processed food, insulin resistance has become a key risk factor for blood sugar imbalance during pregnancy.

Vitamin D

Vitamin D deficiencies are epidemic in all age groups, due to inadequate intake and lack of sun exposure. Vitamin D enhances the absorption of calcium, reduces bone breakdown, and prevents softening of the bone. Vitamin D receptors have been identified in almost every tissue and cell in the body. Vitamin D is involved in regulating cell growth and maturation, stimulating insulin release from the pancreas, and modulating the function of immune cells. It also supports estrogen production in women, and low levels are linked with infertility. Children born to mothers deficient in vitamin D while pregnant show lower bone masses and growth at age 10. Low levels have also been linked with low birth weight. Low serum vitamin D levels have been found with gestational diabetes and may be a good lab indicator of insulin resistance. Supplementing with Vitamin D and calcium together optimizes glucose metabolism. Low vitamin D levels in the first trimester are linked with a twofold increase of preeclampsia later in pregnancy.

Zinc

Zinc has many roles in the body; however, its role in cell division and cell repair is the most important for proper growth of the baby. Zinc deficiency in humans has been linked to reduced growth rates and developmental delays during both pregnancy and breastfeeding. Low levels are linked with increased pregnancy complications, such as preeclampsia, prolonged labors, and vaginal bleeding. In males, zinc is involved with making sperm and for normal sexual development. Zinc also positively affects insulin signaling and glucose uptake into the cells.

Additional Tips

Your first steps for a healthy pregnancy are to start a healthy pregnancy diet, exercise, boost your antioxidant and nutrient intake, and lower homocysteine levels. Here are some additional things to think about for each pregnancy complication we have discussed:

Preterm Labor

Preterm labor is defined as delivery before 36 weeks of pregnancy. Here are some key ways to prevent it:

Strengthen the membranes. About 40 percent of preterm labor is caused by premature rupture of membranes. Magnesium, copper, and vitamin C are linked to the biochemical processes that maintain the strength of the membranes. Vitamin C is specifically involved with collagen synthesis, an important aspect of healthy membranes.

Lengthen the pregnancy with essential fatty acids. DHA found in fish oil and eggs has been shown to lengthen pregnancy by four to seven days. Although that may not sound like a lot, every day is precious for infant development and decreasing the risk of complications for the newborn.

Reduce risk of infection. Fresh fruit, berry juice, and fermented milk products containing probiotics decrease the risk of urinary tract infections, a risk factor for early delivery. I recommend boosting your immune system with vitamins C and E, as well as probiotics. Avoid things that suppress the immune system, like white sugar, and be sure to increase spices in your diet for their antimicrobial effects.

Normalize iron levels. Iron deficiency and iron overload have both been linked with pre-term labor so low dose iron supplementation is a safe choice.

Gestational Diabetes

Lack of blood sugar control increases the risk of complications to the baby (higher rate of miscarriage, birth defects, low blood sugar at birth, and high birth weight) and to the mother (preterm labor, preeclampsia, and high blood pressure). There also may be a possible risk increase of 35 to 50 percent of developing type 2 diabetes within 16 years of being diagnosed with gestational diabetes. Pregnancy is a time when we get a window into the pancreas to see how we are doing with our blood sugar management. The best ways to prevent gestational diabetes are:

Get tested early. Treatment is more effective if started early. The test for gestational diabetes is traditionally done at 28 weeks of pregnancy, but better results are obtained if you are tested at 24 weeks.

Stabilize blood sugar levels. It is important to stabilize blood sugar by eating small meals frequently so your blood sugar does not crash. Increase fiber and always eating a carb with protein or fat as they take longer to digest. This will increase the absorption time of sugar from your digestive tract to your blood. The Nurse's Health study found for every 10 grams of fiber added the risk of gestational diabetes drops by 26 percent.

Say no to fruit juice and pop. Sugar is rapidly absorbed into the bloodstream when it is not paired with fiber. Soda pop and fruit drinks are associated with an increased risk of diabetes. Get your hydration from water and water-rich vegetables instead. Cut back on high-starch veggies such as corn and potatoes.

Make your lifestyle changes before pregnancy. The Nurses' Health study showed that risk of gestational diabetes was lower in women who ate a diet high in fruit, green leafy veggies, poultry, and fish before pregnancy compared with those who ate the typical Western diet of red and processed meats, refined grains, sweets, French fries, and pizza. Those who exercised regularly reduced their risk by 23 percent. Women at the highest risk were those who watched 20 hours or more of television a week.

Get some vitamin D from the sun. Vitamin D deficiency has been linked with insulin resistance. Get more sun while going easy on your skin by going outside without sunscreen for 20 minutes three times per week, avoiding peak times of the day.

Sprinkle with cinnamon. Cinnamon may augment the action of insulin. One-half teaspoon daily is recommended.

Take chromium and biotin. Research shows that 600 mcg of chromium picolinate and 2 mg of biotin per day improve blood sugar control and lower cholesterol and triglycerides. Chromium combined with zinc has a positive effect on insulin signaling and glucose uptake into the cells.

Preeclampsia

Preeclampsia is a pregnancy complication marked by severe high blood pressure and elevated protein in the urine. It's an emergency situation, and if it's not treated quickly, it can be fatal for both mother and infant. We don't understand exactly what causes it, but we do know there are some ways to help prevent it.

Correct calcium and magnesium deficiencies. Women with calcium and magnesium deficiency and those at high risk of developing preeclampsia benefit from supplementation.

Cut the trans fats. Diets higher in trans fatty acids are associated with increased risk of preeclampsia. Trans fats are mainly found in partially hydrogenated vegetable oils and processed foods. Read labels carefully and avoid foods that contain trans fats.

Supplement with essential fatty acids starting before conception or in the first trimester. Preeclampsia is associated with pathological changes to the placenta in the first trimester. Large amounts of essential fatty acids may be needed to maintain the cell membranes of the placenta.

Increase your fiber. Women who consume more than 24 grams of fiber per day can cut their risk of pre-eclampsia in half.

Fight free radicals. According to the Preeclampsia Study, taking 400 IU of vitamin E and 1,000 mg of vitamin C reduced the incidence of this disease in high-risk women. Researchers are looking into whether correlation exists between high homocysteine levels and free radicals that could contribute to the damage of the lining of the blood vessels and cause increased blood pressure. This is important because if they're not independent risk factors, both issues need to be addressed at the same time.

Chapter Five
Key Supplements to Consider

I recommend that pregnant women take food-based supplements, if possible as they are closer to nature versus being synthetic. For safety concerns, it is important to start with lower doses. The use of larger doses of vitamin and minerals, should be in consultation with a health care professional who will assess if the lab work or clinical picture indicates it is necessary. Whenever possible, I use liquid supplements because they are better absorbed. The brand I most frequently recommend is Floradix. Unlike tablets or capsules, liquids do not require any breakdown by the digestive tract for absorption. Liquids can spread out over more absorption sites in the digestive tract, further aiding absorption.

Prenatal Multivitamin And Mineral Supplement With Folic Acid

Simply taking a high-quality multivitamin/multimineral while you are pregnant has significant benefits to both you and your baby. It reduces the incidence of high blood pressure in the mother, childhood cancers, and birth defects. It provides a broad spectrum of nutrients to prevent deficiencies. If homocysteine levels are elevated, additional B6, B12, and folic acid in a B complex should also be taken.

Antioxidants

Antioxidant nutrients are useful for preventing pregnancy complications, such as miscarriage, preeclampsia, preterm labor, and gestational diabetes. Additional vitamin E (400 IU) and up to 1,000 mg vitamin C may be helpful. I like using concentrates of the dark pigmented berries with Masquelier's Original OPCs from grape seeds in a product from Flora called Grape Seed Extract Plus (or Beyond Grape Seed in Canada).

Floradix Liquid Iron And Herbs

In one study involving pregnant women, liquid ferrous gluconate (a form of iron) was compared to other liquid and solid iron supplements. It was effective at lower dosages in treating iron deficiency and anemia. The liquid was also better tolerated, without the side effects, such as digestive upset, found in the other groups.

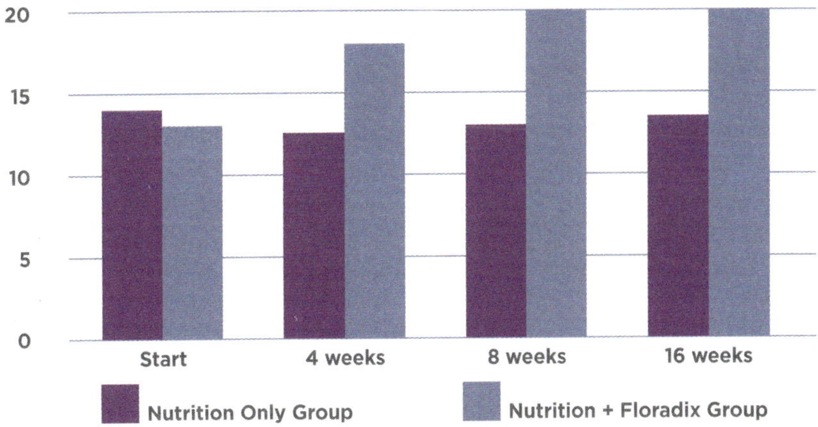

Floradix Studies

Floradix Iron and Herbs is designed for prevention and treatment of iron deficiency. The absorption rate of iron ferrous gluconate in Floradix Iron and Herbs Liquid was tested at the University of Munich's Medical Centre by means of radioactively tagged iron. The absorption rate was shown to be nearly 25 percent compared to 12 percent absorption of ferrous sulfate tables, which is the most commonly prescribed iron. The ferrous sulfate tablets were also poorly tolerated. One of the most common side effects of this form of iron is constipation.

In a 2002 study on Floradix at the Heidelberg Women's University Clinic, Floradix Iron and Herbs was effective at raising serum ferritin levels and 90 percent of the participants were able to take it without side affects, including constipation. The study also showed that 70 percent of the women reported improved symptoms after taking Floradix, compared with 28 percent who just increased intake of iron-rich foods.

One of the things I like best about Floradix is the way it is made. Ferrous gluconate, one of the most absorbable forms of iron, is combined with brewer's yeast. The iron is incorporated into the yeast cell wall, further enhancing its absorption. Rosehips, B vitamins, and vitamin C are added to aid absorption and help make red blood cells. Herbs and foods rich in iron such as spinach, nettles, and kelp, along with herbs that stimulate digestive enzymes, are also part of this unique formulation.

Liquid Calcium And Magnesium Supplements And Vitamin D

In addition to Floradix iron, I recommend Floradix Calcium-Magnesium, and vitamin D. I prefer the highly absorbable forms of calcium such as calcium gluconate, lactate, and citrate; for magnesium, I recommend magnesium gluconate and citrate. Taking your supplement at bedtime can help prevent or relieve leg cramps, which are common during pregnancy.

Probiotics

Since the mother provides the organisms to kick-start the gut flora for her baby, the healthier strains she has in her digestive and reproductive tracts, the healthier start the baby will have in life. Probiotics used in pregnancy and breastfeeding have been shown to improve the immunoprotection of breast milk and significantly reduce eczema in the first two years of life in both allergic and non-allergic mothers. I recommend Udo's Choice Bifido Plus (in Canada, Udo's Choice Hi-Potency Bowel Probiotic).

Essential Fatty Acids

DHA, an omega-3 fatty acid, taken during pregnancy and breastfeeding has been shown to increase infant IQ, improve social behavior, improve vision and hearing, and reduce risk of eczema. In the pregnant mother, it is useful in preventing preterm labor and preeclampsia. DHA levels in pregnant women decline throughout pregnancy. This may mean that the mother cannot meet the high requirement of the growing baby without supplementation.

Supplementing with fish oil by itself can reduce the amount of omega-6 essential fatty acids (GLA & arachidonic acid) in the body. Arachidonic acid is crucial for infant brain development, and GLA ensures sufficient birth weight. In a double-blind, randomized, placebo-controlled trial, Efanatal, a combination of fish oil and Efamol Evening Primrose Oil (omega 6), was found to increase DHA and GLA without reducing arachidonic acid levels. The *Journal of Nutritional Science and Vitaminology* studied women taking Efamol Evening Primrose Oil over an eight-month period while breastfeeding. The fat content of the breast milk was 15 percent higher in those taking Efamol Evening Primrose Oil versus a decline of 23 percent in the placebo group. Efamol Evening Primrose Oil is derived from the most biologically active varieties of the plant and is gently extracted to maintain the integrity of the oil.

Final Thoughts

Being pregnant can be the most significant time in a woman's life. To take the worry out of getting and staying pregnant, focus should be placed on a healthful diet, health-promoting lifestyle, and dietary supplements when appropriate. Pregnant women should exercise caution when using dietary supplements. Be sure to work closely with your health care professional regarding supplement usage.

Selected References

Adzersen KH, et al. Examination of the effectiveness of Floradix (liquid) in women with a low ferritin level- a prospective, random, open intervention study. Department of Gynecology, Endocrinology, and Fertility disorders, Heidelberg Women's University Clinic. 2002.

Bodnar LM, et al. Maternal vitamin D deficiency increases the risk of preeclampsia. *Journal of Clinical Endocrinology and Metabolism* May 2007.

Cant A, et al. The effect of maternal supplementation with linoleic and gamma-linolenic acid on the fat composition and content of human milk: A Placebo Controlled Trial. *Journal of Nutritional Science and Vitaminology* 37: 573-579, 1991.

Carr CA. Evidence Based Diabetes Screening During Pregnancy. *Journal of Midwifery and Women's Health*, May/June 46(3): 152-158, 2001.

Casanueva E, et al. Vitamin C supplementation to prevent premature rupture of the chorioamniotic membranes: a randomized trial. *American Journal of Clinical Nutrition* 81(4):859-863, 2005.

Chavarro, J & W. Willett. *The Fertility Diet*. New York: McGraw Hill, 2008.

Chavarro J, et al, Iron Intake and Risk of Ovulatory Infertility. *Obstetrics & Gynecology* 108(5):1145-52, 2006.

Chittumma P, et al. Comparison of the effectiveness of ginger and B6 for treatment of nausea and vomiting in early pregnancy: a randomized double blind controlled trial. *Journal of the Medical Association of Thailand* 90(1):15-20, 2007.

Cnattingius S, et al. Caffeine Intake and the Risk of First Trimester Spontaneous Abortion. *New England Journal of Medicine* 343: 1839-45, 2001.

Cogswell M, et al. Iron supplementation during pregnancy, anemia, and birth weight: a randomized controlled trial. *American Journal of Clinical Nutrition* 78: 773-81, 2003.

de Lorgeril M, et al. Mediterranean diet, traditional risk factors, and the rate of cardiovascular complications after myocardial infarction; final report of the Lyon Diet Heart Study. *Circulation* 99:779-85, 1999.

Geohas J, et al. Chromium Picolinate and Biotin Combination Reduces Atherogenic Index of Plasma in Patients with Type 2 Diabetes Mellitus: A Placebo-Controlled, Double-Blinded, Randomized Clinical Trial. *American Journal of Medical Sciences* 333 (3): 145-153, 2007.

Geppert J, et al. Co-supplementation with evening primrose oil and fish oil does not lower arachidonic acid status and increase the dihomogammalinolenic acid status of women of childbearing age. *British Journal of Nutrition*, June 2008.

Goh YI, et al. Prenatal Multivitamin Supplementation and Rates of Pediatric Cancers: A Meta-Analysis. *Clinical Pharmacology & Therapeutics* 81(5): 685-9, 2007.

Henmi H, et al. Effects of ascorbic acid supplementation on serum progesterone levels in patients with a luteal phase defect. *Fertility and Sterility* 80:459–61, 2003.

Hofmeyr GJ, et al. Dietary calcium supplementation for prevention of pre-eclampsia and related problems: a systematic review and commentary. *British Journal of Obstetrics and Gynecology* 114: 933-43, 2007.

Horvath A, et al. Effect of supplementation of women in high risk pregnancies with long-chain polyunsaturated fatty acids on pregnancy outcomes and growth measures at birth: a meta-analysis of randomized controlled trials. *British Journal of Nutrition* 98(2): 253-259, 2007.

Javaid MK, et al. Maternal vitamin D status during pregnancy and childhood bone mass at age 9 years: a longitudinal study. *Lancet* 367: 36-43, 2006.

Jones G, et al. Maternal diet during pregnancy is associated with bone mineral density in children: a longitudinal study. *European Journal of Clinical Nutrition* 54: 749-756, 2000.

Maconochie N, et al. Risk factors for first trimester miscarriage—results from a UK-population-based case-control study. *British Journal of Obstetrics and Gynecology* 114(2): 170-86, 2006.

Maghbooli Z, et al. Correlation between vitamin D (3) deficiency and insulin resistance in pregnancy. *Diabetes Metabolism Research Review,* July 2, 2007.

Makrides M, et al. Efficacy and tolerability of low-dose iron supplements during pregnancy: a randomized controlled trial. *American Journal of Clinical Nutrition* 78(1):145-53, 2003.

Milman N, et al. Iron status in Danish women, 1984-1994: a cohort comparison of changes in iron stores and the prevalence of iron deficiency and iron overload. *European Journal of Haematology* 71(1): 51-61, 2003.

Parry S and Strauss JF. Premature Rupture of the Fetal Membranes; *New England Journal of Medicine* 338: 663-670, 1998.

Poston L, et al. Vitamin C and vitamin E in pregnant women at risk for preeclampsia (VIP trial): randomized placebo controlled trial. *Lancet* 367(9517): 1145-54, 2006.

Rautava S et al. Probiotics during pregnancy and breast-feeding might confer immunomodulatory protection against atopic disease in the infant. *Journal of Allergy and Clinical Immunology* 109 (1):119-121, 2002.

Ronnenberg A, et al. Preconception homocysteine and B vitamin status and birth outcomes in Chinese women. *American Journal of Clinical Nutrition* 76(6): 385-391, 2002.

Royal College of Obstetricians and Gynecologists Position Statement on Exercise in Pregnancy Issue 4, Feb 2006.

Sattar N, et al. Essential fatty acids in relation to pregnancy complications and fetal development. *British Journal of Obstetrics and Gynecology,* December 105 (12): 1248-1255, 1998.

Seonae Y, et al. Possible Beneficial Effect of Exercise, by Reducing Oxidative Stress, on the Incidence of Preeclampsia. *Journal of Women's Health and Gender Based Medicine* 10(10):983-989, 2001.

Smith C, Crowther C, Beilby J, et al. Acupuncture to Treat Nausea and Vomiting in Early Pregnancy: A Randomized Controlled Trial. *Birth* 29(1):1-9, March 2002.

Toescu V, et al. Changes in plasma lipids and markers of oxidative stress in normal pregnancy and pregnancies complicated by diabetes. *Clinical Science* 106:93-98, 2004.

Velzing-Aarts FV, et al. Plasma choline and betaine and their relation to plasma homocysteine in normal pregnancy. *The American Journal of Clinical Nutrition* 81(6), 1383-1389, 2005.

Ward N, et al. Study of Preconceptual Care and Pregnancy. *Journal of Nutritional & Environmental Medicine* 5:205-208, 1995.

Zhang C, Liu S, et al. Dietary Fiber intake, dietary glycemic load, and the risk of gestational diabetes mellitus. *Diabetes Care* 29 (10): 2223-30, 2006.

Zhang C, Solomon CG, et al. A prospective study of pregravid physical activity and sedentary behaviors in relation to the risk for gestational diabetes mellitus. *Archives of Internal Medicine* 166(5): 543-8, 2006.

Zhang C, et al. Vitamin C and the Risk of Gestational Diabetes: A Case Controlled Study. *Journal of Reproductive Medicine,* April 49(4): 257-66, 2004.

For more information about the products mentioned, visit:

www.florahealth.com